ooh la la!

perfect body

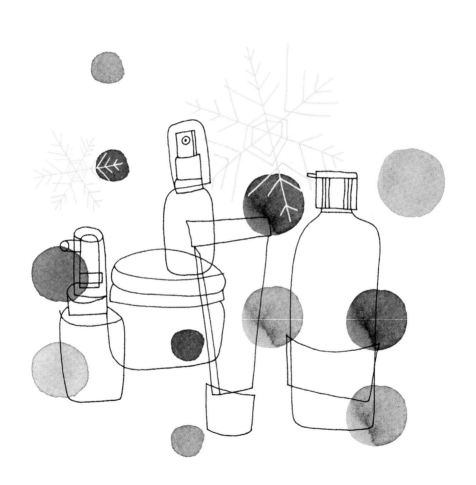

ooh la la!
perfect body

Susie Galvez

Illustrated by Chico Hayasaki

MQP

Published by MQ Publications Limited
12 The Ivories
6–8 Northampton Street
London, N1 2HY
email: mail@mqpublications.com
website: www.mqpublications.com

Copyright © MQ Publications Limited 2004
Text copyright © Susie Galvez 2004

Illustrator: Chico Hayasaki/www.cwc-i.com
Editor: Laura Kesner
Senior Designer: Victoria Bevan

ISBN: 1-84072-537-0
10 9 8 7 6 5 4 3 2 1

All rights reserved. No part of this publication may be used or reproduced or transmitted in any form or by any means, electronic or mechanical, including photocopy, recording, or any information storage and retrieval system now known or to be invented without permission in writing from the publishers.

This book is intended as an informational guide only and is not to be used as a substitute for professional medical care or treatment. Neither the author nor the publisher can be held responsible for any damage, injury, or otherwise resulting from the use of the information in this book.

Printed and bound in France by *Partenaires-Livres*® (JL)

Contents

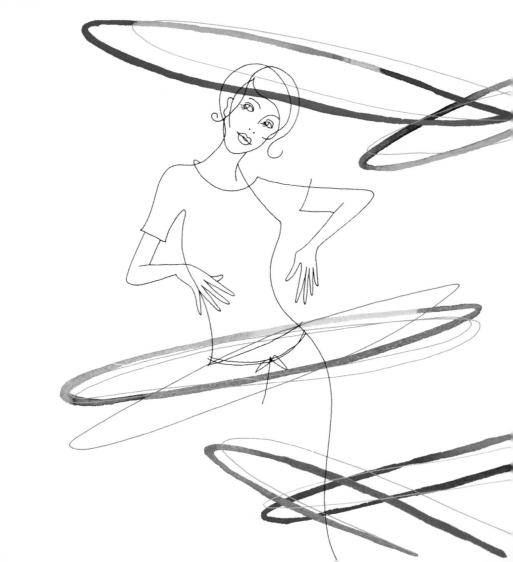

Introduction

Many of us spare no expense in caring for all those ultra-special outfits hanging in our closets. However, we completely neglect the most extraordinary thing we possess—our bodies.

It's time to take a look at your body's "care instructions" label!

Containing 101 must-have beauty tips, *Ooh La La! Perfect Body* fills you in on everything you need to know about giving your body the care it deserves, inside and out.

Feel fabulous in no time with secrets from the world's top spas. Find out how to fix pesky beauty breakers in a flash. Revitalize with your own private bathing getaway. Get gorgeous hands and feet with salon-savvy TLC.

From head to toe, *Ooh La La! Perfect Body* has tips for keeping every single inch of your body smooth, supple, and in just puuurrrfect condition. Ooh La La!

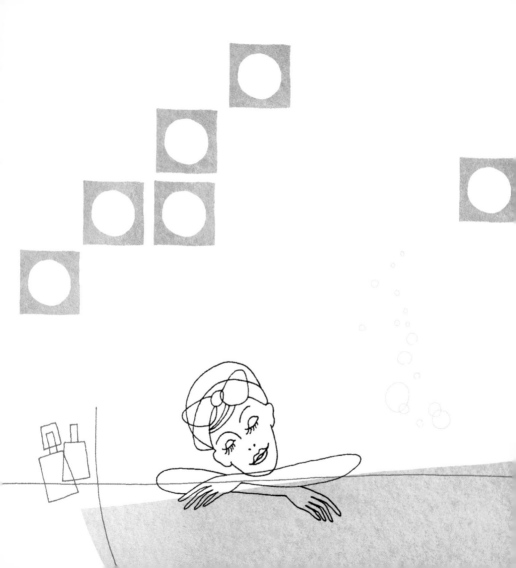

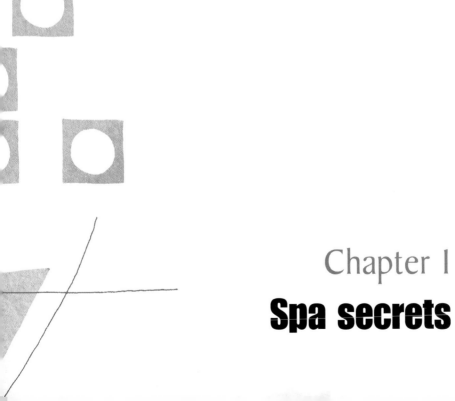

Chapter 1

Spa secrets

Smooth operator

Dry brushing, although ancient in origin, is a super-modern way to keep dry, flaky skin away for good. Use a natural-fiber bath brush that has a handle attachment to reach your back area. Before bathing, while skin is dry, begin dry brushing at the toes, feet, ankles, and legs. Work up the body, always in the direction of the heart. Continue up the torso, stomach, back, and arms. All it takes is about five to seven gentle, long brush strokes over each area. Allow the motion to do the work—gentle brushing is best. The movement is similar to that of shaving. Start dry brushing two or three times a week until your skin begins to feel very soft to the touch. To maintain softness, dry brush once a week. Shower as usual after brushing, pat dry, and add a bit of moisture. You will find that you actually use less moisturizer as time goes on. This is because the skin will be more efficient at producing it from the inside.

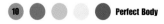

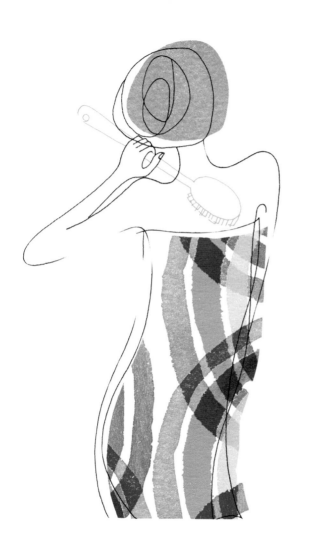
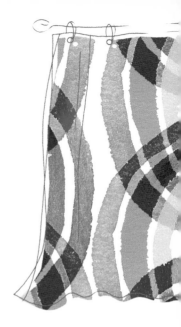

Rub-a-dub-dub

For an all-over, spring-back-to-life feeling, grab a towel. Instead of the same old pat dry after showering, briskly rub your entire body with a terry cloth towel. The rubbing back and forth creates a warming friction and revives even the most tired skin. Your skin will feel alive, your circulation will be in high gear, and you will glow all over!

Material girl

Exfoliating materials come in an array of different sources. Washcloths are the gentlest exfoliators—the only kind gentle enough for delicate facial skin. Loofahs, sea sponges, silk hand mitts, and soaps containing exfoliating products such as oatmeal, seaweed, or crushed almonds are all excellent in removing dead skin from the body. Remember to let the material do the work. Be gentle—go easy.

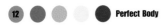

Off with the old, in with the new

To rid the skin of extra dry, flaky cells and replenish moisture at the same time, try this spa favorite. Mix two tablespoons of Dead Sea salt and one cup of olive oil. Shower as usual, then while still in the shower, gently rub the body with the mixture. Rinse, and rinse again. Rub any remaining oil into the skin and pat dry. The Dead Sea salt contains minerals that will help loosen dead skin while the olive oil, with its monounsaturated fat, will moisturize and soften.

Introduce yourself

While baths are a wonderful way to relax and de-stress, they are also wonderful for getting to know your skin. From the neck up, we know our skin like the back of our hands, but body skin often goes unnoticed—or worse—forgotten. Take time to introduce yourself to you. Check out your body skin with as much care as you do your face. A sure way to love yourself is to take care of your body and enjoy your uniqueness. Polish and smooth the skin, slather on body cream, and gently pat on a luxurious body powder that says, "I am special, and I enjoy who I am."

Cheers!

Planning a special night out? Set the mood beforehand. Indulge in a pink champagne bath. Add two cups of pink champagne, two capfuls of an enriching bubble bath, two teaspoons of olive oil and $\frac{1}{4}$ cup of sea salt. Light a couple of candles, pour yourself a glass of the pink champagne, and soak. Gently dry off and apply your favorite moisturizer, powder, and perfume.

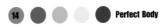

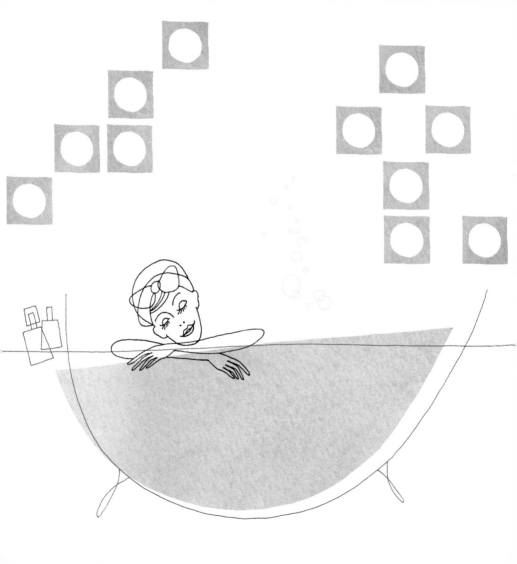

Nix at night

Dry brushing should be done during the morning, since it stimulates the circulatory system. Brushing at night could keep you up and disturb sleep—unless you need to be stimulated for a night out on the town, then a quick dry brush before preparing to party may be just what you need. Don't say I didn't warn you.

Get away

Day spas are all the rage right now. From a facial or a massage, to a pedicure or a manicure, day spas are the place to go for a professional body treatment. The difference between a "day" spa and a "stay" spa is that you go home after receiving your treatment at the day spa. A stay spa is usually tied to a resort or special destination hotel. While sounding wonderful, a stay spa requires planning, travel, time off, etc. A day spa offers the same luxuries, but allows you to schedule an hour or a day without extensive traveling. Both have their place, but don't wait until your vacation to indulge in a skin-affirming treatment. Visit your local day spa today!

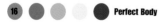

Mud pack

The ultimate body rejuvenation is a mud treatment. Europeans believe that a mud treatment not only softens and removes dead skin, but also soothes tired muscles and relieves itchy skin. One way to "take the cure" is to immerse yourself in a vat of mud from a mineral spring. Great if you can find it. The other option is to have a mud treatment applied at the spa. Mud is brushed onto the skin, and you are wrapped

in a plastic cocoon until the mud cures; or at home you can slather yourself with Dead Sea mud product and sit in the bathroom until the mud dries—then wash it off. If you are doing this treatment at home, invest in a small plastic stool on which you can sit while the treatment works. Cleaning up will be a breeze as you can wash yourself and the stool in the shower. Then pat yourself dry and add moisturizer.

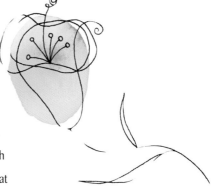

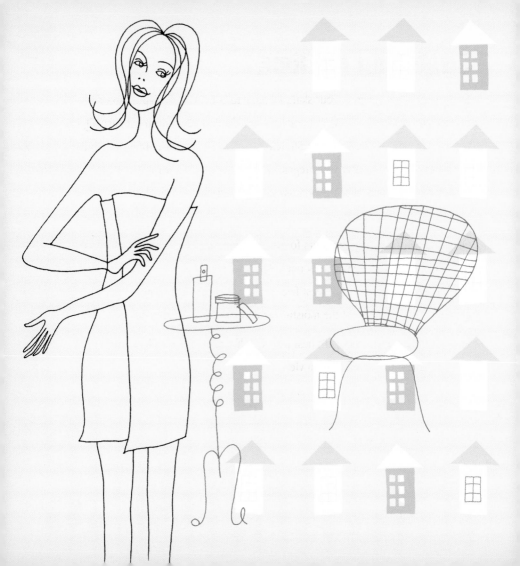

Stretching the limit

Stretch marks are a sign of your skin's inability to cope with the rapid expansion of flesh underneath the area. The collagen and elastin fibers underneath actually tear with the sheer strain of it all. Stretch marks usually appear in times of rapid weight gain, such as puberty or pregnancy. They are very red when they first appear, but over time (thank goodness) they will fade away to an almost unnoticeable silvery shade.

Once you get them, they are yours forever. However, keeping the skin well moisturized can help prevent new ones. Apply a body moisturizer after every bath or shower, and give it at least five minutes to absorb before putting on clothing. This ensures that the moisturizer's goodness has time to penetrate.

Suntans are a stretch mark gal's best friend. Self-tanners are excellent cover-ups for disguising the marks from view.

Rosy glow

Cherries are full of malic acid—perfect for a quick body glow treatment. Malic acid speeds up cell removal and helps with skin exfoliating. Malic acid is one of the fruit acids often used in professional treatments. Mix three tablespoons of cherry juice concentrate with two tablespoons of sea salt. Dampen skin in the shower and lightly apply mixture to the entire body. You will only need to rub gently, as the fruit acids do all the hard work for you. Rinse thoroughly and moisturize to rehydrate the skin. Your body will feel fresh and clean, and give off a healthy glow.

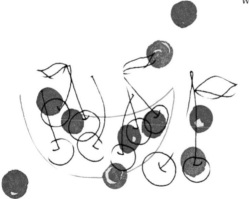

Inexpensive indulgence

Hands down, a manicure is one of the most inexpensive ways to indulge. A professional nail technician will clip, file, and correct nail length and shape, remove or soften cuticles, hydrate hands, and polish to perfection in less than one hour. Yet you will feel as if you have escaped for much longer. A weekly manicure can do wonders not only for your nails, but also for your mental state.

Hands are always on display and speak volumes about you without saying a word. If a weekly professional pampering session is out of the budget, at least plan to enjoy a professional manicure every four to six weeks and maintain your nails at home between visits. The professional will be able to correct the shape and ensure that the nail bed remains healthy and the nails remain strong.

Give 'em the brush off

A natural bristle nailbrush is wonderful for cleaning under nails. It also helps keep cuticles in check by removing dead skin cells. If your nail area is on the tender side, use a soft bristle toothbrush to gently cleanse the area. Store with your nail implements and use daily.

Don't be stingy

While in most cases a little dab of a skin care product will do, sunscreen is different. Slather it on liberally for the best protection. This is the one product where more is best. Being skimpy with sunscreen means that you are apt to miss areas. If you apply a thinner layer, your SPF of 15 will not absorb effectively and will only have the protection value of an SPF of 8 or less. Remember your sunscreen is moving with you, so apply extra to the high-traffic areas on your body such as hands, feet, and any area where garments, glasses, or sunhats could wear it off.

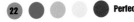

A leg up

Varicose veins can show up at any time. There are several causes for their occurrence: heredity (if your mother has them, be extra careful); weight gain or loss; and restricted movement, such as sitting or standing for extended periods of time.

To keep ahead of varicosities, begin a walking program to get the blood flowing. Eating a high-fiber, vegetable-rich diet with plenty of water will also help reduce and/or prevent the unsightly veins from appearing.

If you are troubled by varicosities, try sleeping with the feet raised: place a two to four inch block under each of the feet at the bottom of the bed. (Bonus—elevation is great for facial skin too!) Also, be sure to uncross your legs every time you catch yourself doing so. Never sit for more than one hour without moving around—if only to walk around the office or kitchen for a couple of minutes.

Lycra hosiery is excellent for keeping the vein compressed and aiding circulation around the legs. And thank goodness! They are now virtually undetectable from regular hosiery.

Gam glam

To show off toned and self-tanned legs, use a body moisturizer that contains shimmering ingredients such as gold or bronze flecks. Tanning salons often carry these products for their clients to show off their tan. Your golden glow will be enhanced by the sparkle. Try blending some of the product along your shin bones to give a sexy sheen and to create the illusion of slimmer legs.

Concoct a quick at-home version by mixing a bit of hair shine product with a little bit of shimmery face powder and apply to legs.

Fake bake

The safest tan comes out of a bottle. To enjoy your fake bake longer, use a body scrub before tanning to remove excess flaky skin that would otherwise soak up the color and create a patchy finish. Shave your legs. Massage body lotion on all areas to be treated. This will combat any dry areas and produce a smooth surface on which to apply the self-tanner.

If you have a choice, go with a light shade. You can always go darker, but it is almost impossible to lighten up after applying.

Remember, less is more. Start in small sections, using long broad strokes to avoid streaks and uneven areas. After you have finished applying, go back and clean areas that are not usually exposed to the sun, such as armpits, nipples, soles of feet, and between the fingers.

Reapply weekly to keep the fake bake going all season long.

Flake off

Exfoliation is about much more than just removing dead skin cells and everyday dirt. Exfoliation increases blood flow to the skin and helps your circulatory and lymphatic systems to release toxins. Removing the extra dead skin also aids in reducing the occurrence of ingrown hairs. Plus, once the extra cells are gone, moisturizers will absorb better. Say bye-bye to flakiness and itchiness.

Exfoliating is easy to do. Simply keep a loofah or mesh sponge in the shower along with a gentle exfoliating shower gel. Once or twice a week, while your hair is conditioning, apply a small amount of scrub to your loofah or mesh sponge and go over the body. Rinse well. Be sure to moisturize afterward to rehydrate the skin.

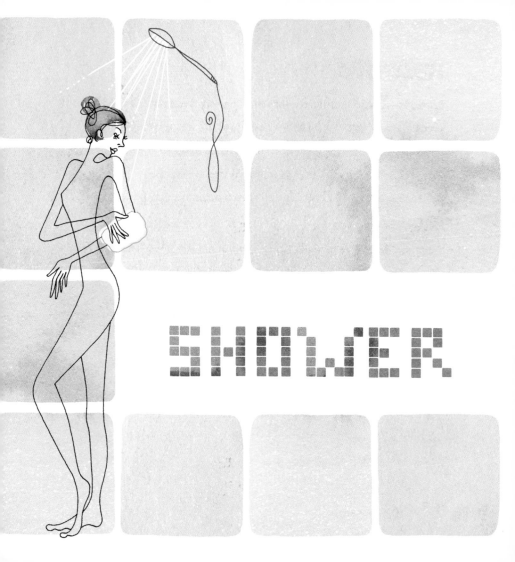

SHOWER

Under the sea

Seaweed is a popular spa cure. It is popular because not only does it stimulate the metabolism, but it also contains marine nutrients and botanicals found only in the sea.

You can purchase seaweed bath soaks for an at-home spa detoxifying treatment. After soaking in the seaweed solution for 15 minutes, rinse off, and pat dry. Roll yourself in a blanket to rest for ten to 15 minutes and allow the body to process the treatment. Since seaweed is such a powerful detoxifier, the treatment could leave you a bit lightheaded. Be sure to rest and recover.

Poetic waxing

Waxing is a great way to remove hair for weeks at a time. However, due to the extra exfoliating effect of waxing, be careful of waxed areas when traveling to the beach or anyplace where you are more likely to be exposed to the sun. Your best bet is to confine waxing of legs, bikini line, and underarms to at least four days prior to any sun exposure.

 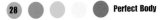 Perfect Body

Wish you were here

Relive your fun-in-the-sun vacation or create a mini vacation anytime you want. Take a luxurious Dead Sea salt bath soak. Afterward, instead of the usual moisturizer, opt for your favorite sunscreen lotion. The smell of the sunscreen will remind you of sunshine and sea breezes. Put on your favorite beach cover up, lie down, close your eyes, breathe deeply, and imagine the islands.

Buy some time

Depilatory creams allow you to go up to two weeks without stubble. But they are not as quick as shaving. The creams need to work on the hair anywhere from 15 to 20 minutes, and are always on the smelly side. However, to forgo the shaving routine for two weeks, it can be worth the wait. Be sure to check for sensitivity and read the label for other precautions. Two weeks razor-less, to say it again, has definite advantages!

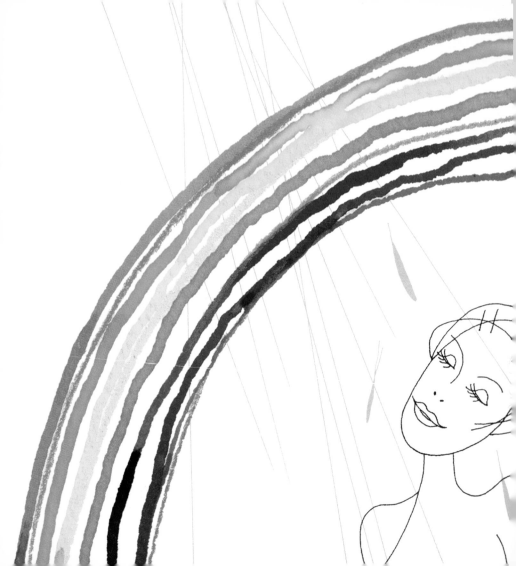

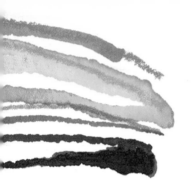

Chapter 2

A good soaking

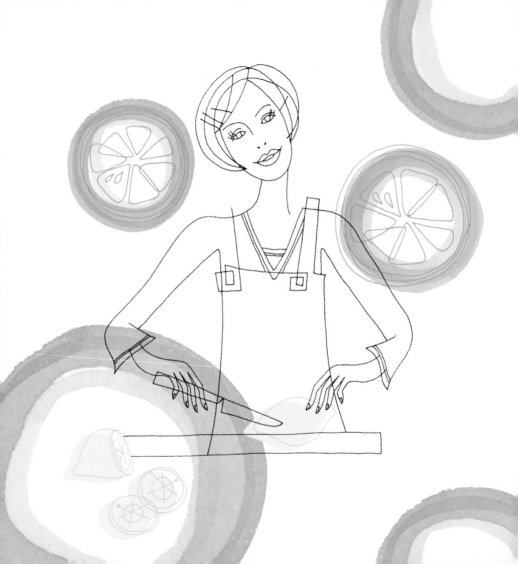

Not just for breakfast

Grapefruit is a natural acid treatment. It is found in high-end products and spa treatments around the world. To experience a world-class spa treatment at home, cut a grapefruit in half and dip it in sugar. Gently rub the entire half over the body. Add more sugar if needed. The grapefruit and sugar combination will revitalize the body, remove excess skin, and leave the body feeling refreshed and revived. What a wake-up call!

When life gives you lemons

Take a soothing lemon soak! Slice a fresh lemon into thin slices and sprinkle over a tub of warm water. Immerse yourself in the wonderful aroma. Lemons contain citrus acid, which is an excellent dead skin remover. The juice aids in gently cleansing the skin while the oil from the lemon rind softly hydrates. This is an excellent cure for sunburned skin as well.

Unappealing

"Orange peel" skin, like the kind of skin that usually appears on the upper arms, is due to poor circulation. Increase circulation in this area by applying a good body scrub as well as using a loofah or scrubbing mitt daily while bathing or showering. Using circular motions, gently but thoroughly cleanse and scrub the area. Be sure to apply an AHA-based (alpha hydroxy acid) moisturizer afterward to continue the exfoliating process. Diligent care will produce sleeker, less bumpy areas.

Breast buddy

Breast self-examination is something that we can do as easily as taking a shower. In fact, while soaping up in the shower, during the week after the end of your period, take time to check your breasts.

* Raise your right arm above your head, and feel the entire breast and armpit using the fingers of your left hand. Make small circles, applying firm pressure, checking for any lumps or hardened areas. Repeat on the other side.

* Hold your right arm up and place your hand on the back of your neck. Check the areas again using small circles while applying firm pressure.

If you detect something that does not feel right, don't panic. Just call your doctor to make an appointment and get it checked out. Remember—be your own breast buddy, and check yourself every single month.

Castaway

Luxury soaps such as hand-milled, triple-milled, and essential oil scented soaps are usually very generous in size. To keep from washing away and wasting any of this well-deserved luxury, cut the soap bar in half with a sharp knife. The smaller size will be easier to hold in the hands and is less likely to get lost in a puddle of water in the soap dish.

Another good idea is to purchase a soap drainer on which to store your luxury soap. This will keep the soap-melting water away and allow the soap to linger longer.

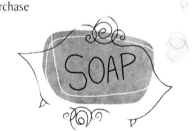

Clean act

A good soap is like a breath of fresh air. It should leave the skin feeling clean and fresh but not taut. Tight skin after washing will mean that you have stripped it of moisture. The skin should feel hydrated after lathering up, without feeling oily. The best choices are milled, vegetable-based soaps. The fragrances are as varied as our moods. A great wake-up soap is one that is scented with a rosemary or citrus fragrance, to invigorate the senses, and prepare you for the day ahead.

Relaxing soaps are those scented with lavender or vanilla, to comfort and calm. Pick a soap to match your mood.

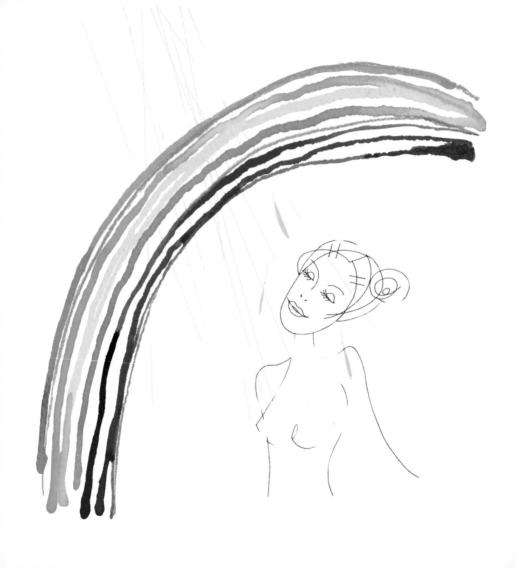

Global warming

Keep your bath or shower water at about 80°F. Any warmer and water will only drain your energy. Any colder and your heart may begin to race.

Overly warm water will remove too much of the skin's natural sebum which helps to keep the skin moisturized. As a good rule, keep bath soaking down to 20 minutes. You will just have to finish reading your novel once you are out and dry. Oversoaking will only deplete your body of water and skin oils, which is the very thing that you are trying to avoid.

Scrub-a-dub

A quick splash under a faucet will not wash when cleaning the hands. Slow down, take your time to moisten, lather, get under the nails, and rinse. The time spent washing the hands should be about 30 seconds. That is about the time it takes to sing the song "Row, Row, Row Your Boat," twice but not out loud—please!

Taking the cure

Thalassotherapy, which features treatments using seawater, has been around for centuries, but is now the current trend in spa treatments. For almost nothing, you can create a detoxifying, bloat-banishing bath spa treatment that would cost a tidy sum at the spa. Add one cup of Epsom salts to a warm bath. Soak for at least 15 minutes. If the water begins to cool, add more hot water. Epsom salts, like seawater, contain magnesium chloride, which aids in drawing out excess fluids. Be sure to drink plenty of water after this treatment, as water will help to continue flushing your system and will keep the bloating away!

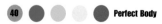

Ankles away

If your ankles tend to swell, try soaking your feet in a bowl of warm water and four tablespoons of Epsom salts to help ease the swelling, as well as soothe tired feet. You can return your telephone calls and read your mail, all while de-puffing your feet!

Tootsie talcum

If you notice that your shoes are wet from sweat when you take them off, put a little powder on the soles of the feet before putting on your shoes and socks. Take extra care when wearing dark-colored hosiery. The last thing you want is visible white powder marks all over your feet and ankles. It is also a good idea to sprinkle talcum powder inside your shoes when you take them off to help absorb any remaining moisture.

In the mood

Candlelight lifts the spirit and calms the soul.
A luxurious bath just would not be complete
without the soft glow of candlelight.
A simple way to keep candles
around is to put up a small
glass shelf over the bath.
The shelf will not take
up much room, and
it will be ready at a
moment's notice. You
will find that any time
is the right time for
the ambience of candles.

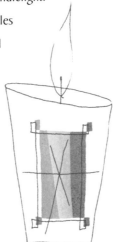

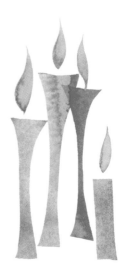

Take it slow

Most of us want hand and body creams that sink in fast. Truth is, the faster absorbing formulas could actually be drying to the skin, since the ingredient included to speed up the process is alcohol.

Choose a slower absorbing formula, without alcohol, for the richest and most nourishing benefits. It will take a minute or two longer, but the longer-term hydrator is well worth the wait.

Firm deal

The newest wave in body creams are ones with firming ingredients in them. While these body formulas, like facial firming creams, temporarily give the look of firm skin—nothing will actually firm the body skin but exercise.

Exercise, and plenty of it, will lessen the lumps and bumps of body skin, giving the outer (and inner) surface a tighter, more toned look and feel.

Close shave

Shaving is still the easiest, cheapest, and most convenient way to remove unwanted hair on the legs and under the arms. To get the closest shave without nicks and cuts, allow the water from the shower or tub to be on the skin at least two minutes prior to shaving. The warm water will soften the area and allow a better shave.

While there are plenty of options on the market, nothing beats the good old disposable razor. Usually they can be purchased in quantity with five or ten in a package. They are great to keep on hand, as you will always have a new one ready and waiting. For extra smoothness, look for razors with a moisturizing strip attached in front of the blade. Used in addition to your shaving gel or soap, a moisturizing strip will help soften the area and leave behind an extra smooth surface.

 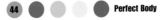

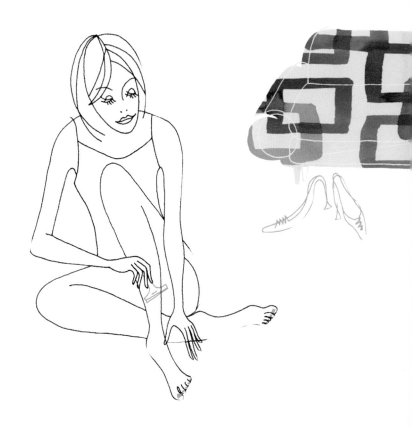

Perfume pizzazz

To add a little pizzazz to your daily dressing routine, spray your favorite fragrance on a few cotton balls. Tuck the perfumed balls into your dresser drawers. A fresh bloom of scent will greet you each time you open the drawer, as well as delicately scenting your garments with your signature aroma. Alternatively, you could always invest in some pretty, scented drawer liners. Lavender bags also make clothes smell delicious. Why not hang some in your wardrobe to keep garments smelling sweet?

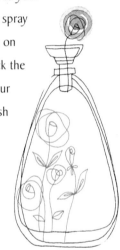

Standing spa appointment

Want to indulge in a spa treatment but only have a couple of minutes? Before you jump in the shower, apply a light coating of body oil, olive oil, or sesame oil to the body. When you are standing in the shower, apply some exfoliation beads or salts directly on the body. Very lightly rub to exfoliate, rinse, and shower as usual. Emerge super soft—super fast! Now that's beauty on the go!

Brief encounters

Want an instant confidence booster—no matter what the occasion? Wear pretty, sexy underwear. Wearing colorful, feminine undergarments creates a mood of confidence and playfulness. Even if no one sees your pretty "undercover" garments, you will know that they are there. Sometimes having a little secret is exactly what you need.

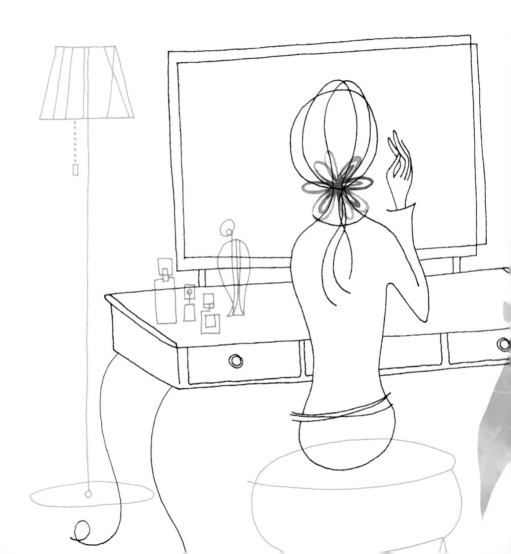

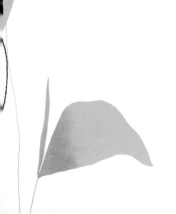

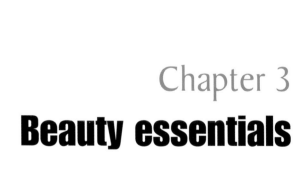

Chapter 3

Beauty essentials

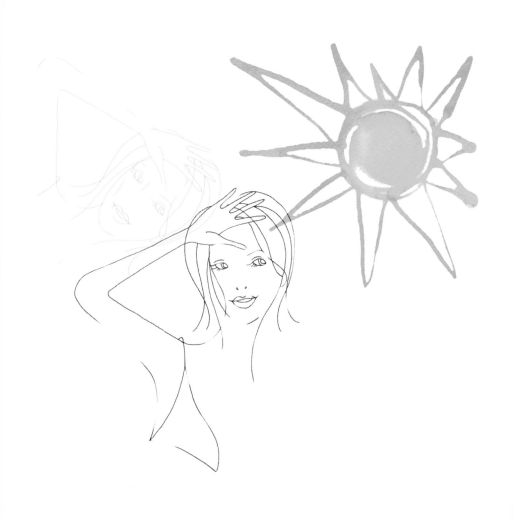

You are my sunshine

Although enough cannot be said about the dangers of excessive sun exposure, did you know that a moderate amount of sunlight, particularly morning sun, is good for your body and mind? Our bodies create vitamin D from exposure to sunlight. In addition, studies show that 15 minutes of indirect sun in the morning will elevate mood and energy levels. Sunlight increases the production of serotonin and norepinephrine, which are natural uppers. The morning sun is best because our eyes are most sensitive to the mood-altering effects of light. So shine on—a tiny bit!

A great way to add a little sunshine to your life is to take a brisk 15-minute walk around your neighborhood each morning. If that is not possible, try opening the curtains as soon as you get up in the morning to welcome in the day as well as the light. If you are lucky enough to have a sunny window in your home, why not enjoy your morning tea or coffee nearby as you greet the day.

Sleeping beauty

The human growth hormone (HGH) is the anti-aging hormone. HGH is responsible for collagen and elastin production, vitality, and skin firmness. It even aids in controlling weight. HGH is released during the seventh and eighth hour of sleep. In addition to helping with all the functions mentioned above, HGH helps repair brain tissue.

Establish a regular bedtime routine that allows you to get the rest your body, as well as your skin needs to perform the millions of functions it does each day. Remember it is really skin, not cotton, that is the fabric of our lives.

Don't pollute — dilute

Too much coffee, tea, or alcohol dehydrates the skin and depletes vitamin B from the body. Vitamin B helps keep nails hard, hair thick, and skin glowing. For every polluting beverage you consume, dilute it by drinking a glass of water.

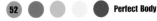

Drink up

Water is the number one source of beautiful skin, without a doubt. Our body is over 70 percent water. Have you ever noticed a water-soaked sponge? It is soft and pliable. What about a dry sponge? It is hard, rough, and rigid. Our skin cells are the same way. Water keeps our cells hydrated and healthy. Drink up this free beauty tip whenever you can, wherever you are. A glass here, a glass there—hopefully it all adds up to eight, eight-ounce glasses or more per day. Without it, no spa treatment or at home treatment will ever do a good job— period. Remember, it is free and it is vital. Drink some now!

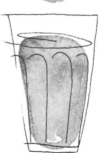

Be your own hobby

If your overall shape is making you unhappy or inhibiting your confidence, maybe it's time to put other pastimes aside and concentrate on your general well-being instead.

Instead of a diet or an exercise program think of this phase of your life as a hobby for a better body. Plan out your body goals, such as weight loss, diet program, and exercise regime.

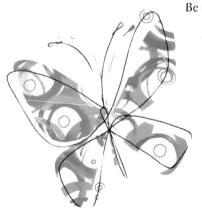

Be completely honest with yourself about what you want: dress size, body shape, time you can devote to achieving goals, and quiet time. Map out a 21 day schedule. Studies show that it takes 21 days to change or create a habit. A healthy "hobby habit" takes planning—so start planning today.

Drive time workout

Next time you are stuck in a traffic jam, put the car in park and test-drive these body toners. Hold each position for 30 seconds, release, and repeat until traffic moves.

✳ Bum tighteners: squeeze glutes tightly while keeping the upper body relaxed.

✳ Bicep boosters: sit with your back flat against the seat, hands holding the bottom of the steering wheel with palms facing up. Contract biceps using the wheel as resistance.

✳ Ab flattener: sit straight up, neck and spine in alignment. Contract ab muscles, pushing belly button toward the spine as if you are trying to get into your tightest jeans.

Traffic jams will never be the same again!

Here kitty

Cats have got it all figured out. They start each day with a slow, whole body stretch that goes from the tips of each toe, up the legs, and onto the torso, ending with a huge yawn. We need to take notes from our feline friends. Stretching first thing in the morning and taking a few deep breaths will allow you to start your morning clearheaded and ready for anything. Meow!

No experience necessary

Walking does not require special training, special clothing, or special equipment—just your two legs. Fitness pros prescribe 30 minutes of steady-paced walking at least four times a week.

In addition to being great exercise, walking is great for the skin since all parts are in motion, moving nutrients and toxins right along. It's also a great stress reliever and re-energizer. It has been said, "You never regret taking a walk, you only regret not taking one." Get up and get moving.

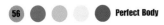

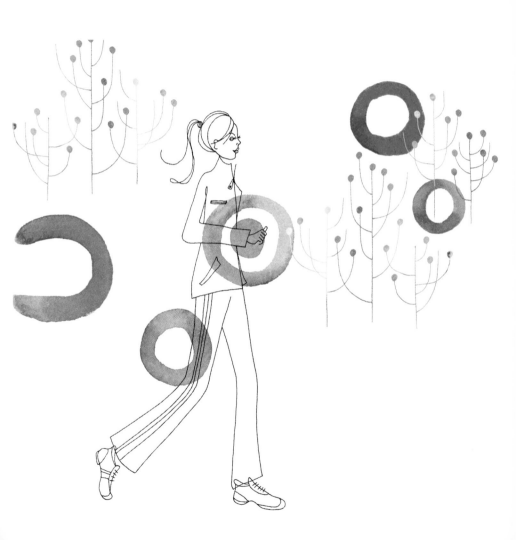

More or less

Losing weight requires meal planning and changed eating habits. To boost the loss even more, combine a balanced weight loss eating plan with regular exercise. Exercise increases the metabolism. If you want to lose more, do more!

Easy street

Your body cannot store fitness, so once you start, you have to keep exercising regularly. Make your routine flexible. If you think it is going to be hard to master, or hard to commit to, don't choose an activity that requires good weather or a long detour from your office or home. Most importantly, you need to enjoy the activity. If you don't, you will always find reasons and excuses to skip it. Find a friend to exercise with, and try to help each other to stay motivated.

Three by five

Invest in a pair of three-pound and five-pound dumbbells. Instead of storing them away for a scheduled exercise session, keep them handy—and noticeable. For a quick pick-me-up, grab the three-pound bells for five minutes of upper bodywork while thinking about what to prepare for dinner, or use the five-pound bells for three minutes during TV commercials.

You will increase your strength and tone without even trying. Also, doing a quick set of reps is a great way to "change gears" from work to arriving home—it can shift your focus and help you to relax. What a great feeling to know that you did something healthy for yourself!

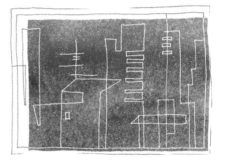

Kid's play

Hulahoops are a great way to relieve stress, appeal to your inner-child, and whittle the waist. If you want a quick waist-whittling exercise instead of the usual ab crunches, try ten minutes of hulahooping. Ten minutes a day for 30 days can take up to two inches off the waist! Instead of a "toy" one, opt for the heavier, bigger kind found at sport stores. Sports model hoops will last longer, and are balanced to give you a smoother and more effective workout. You may want to get an extra hoop, and challenge your friends to a hulahoop contest.

Skipping is also a great way to exercise the whole body. Buy a jump rope from a sport store—a child's jump rope will probably not be long enough for you—and try to skip for about ten minutes a day.

You'll have so much fun, you'll forget you're exercising!

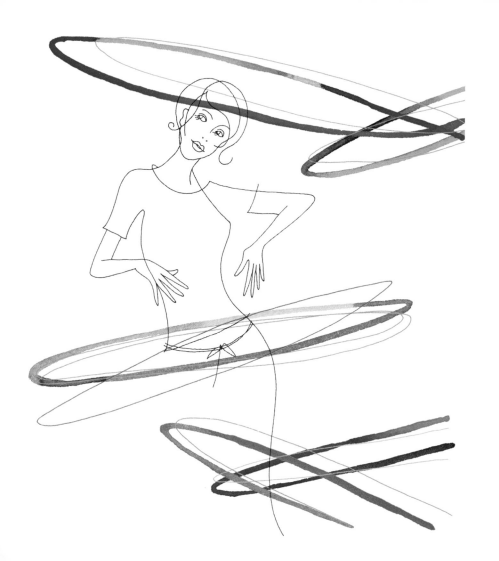

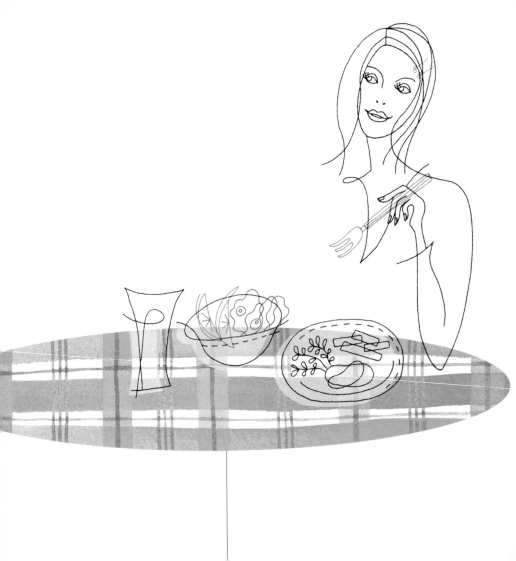

Fat chance

Believe it or not, fat in limited amounts is actually good for the skin. Fat helps the body utilize protein. Fats in oils like olive, corn, sesame, and peanut oil keep the skin supple and hair lustrous. Drizzle some over a fresh green salad or tasty steamed veggies. Enjoy the taste and your beautiful skin.

I am hooked

Most sea fish contains omega-3 fatty acids, which are wonderful for not only the skin and organs, but also for moods and disposition as well. Research shows that a diet rich in omega-3 fatty acids protects the heart and may help to prevent breast cancer. The best catches: mackerel, salmon, halibut, tuna, snapper, and striped bass.

Sugar snack

Sugar is the teeth's enemy. Excess sugar is one of the biggest causes of tooth decay. Try to keep foods tooth-friendly. The best tooth-friendly snacks include:

* Hard cheeses: these are loaded with enamel-strengthening calcium and phosphates.

* Green tea, black tea, and cocoa: these all contain flavonoids and tannins that fight bacteria.

* Spicy and crunchy foods: chilies and crunchy munchies like celery increase saliva production, which fleshes out bits of food and contains bicarbonates to protect against acid and plaque.

 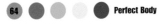

Chew on this

If brushing after lunch or dinner is not possible, chew a piece of sugar-free gum. Sugar-free gum helps to neutralize tooth-attacking acid in the mouth. In addition, chewing sugar-free gum will stimulate the flow of saliva and rub food off the teeth.

For the best post-meal results, try not to end your meal with a sugary dessert. If you simply must have the dessert du jour, slip a piece of sugar-free gum in your mouth after eating to remove the extra sugar you have just consumed. If you don't want to add the extra, empty calories of dessert, pop in a stick of sugar-free gum when the dessert menu is passed around. The sugary taste may suffice as a dessert substitute and help you to resist that sweet treat!

Beauty bite

Keep your smile looking its best by changing your toothbrush as soon as the bristles begin to splay. If you are brushing for two minutes both morning and night as most dentists recommend, three months is the life expectancy for your brush. Keep an extra on hand so you can toss the old brush when the time comes.

Designate space

Find a space that you can dedicate to beauty. Make it a special area just for you, where you can enjoy your daily beauty rituals. Make a place that has everything at your fingertips to allow you to "get it together" with ease. You will instantly feel more organized and more prepared when it comes to beautifying yourself.

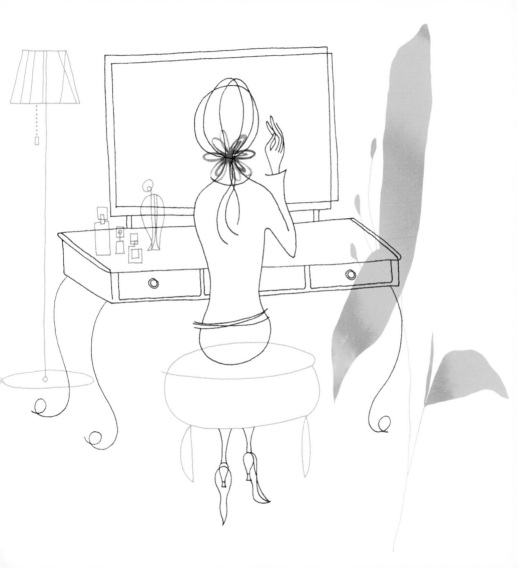

First impressions last

Like it or not, people do judge you by your image. The impression you make can have an enormous effect on how people see you—as an employee, as a potential date, even as a friend. In fact, within just eight seconds, people will make up to eight assumptions about you. From your appearance alone you are judged on socio-economic level; education; trustworthiness; level of sophistication; upbringing; success; moral character; even your future! These impressions are formed by everything about you: your clothes, your posture, your grooming, your attitude, your eye contact—your overall presentation—all create the image you project. If your image is not reflecting the "real" you, make a plan of action and reveal your true self to the world.

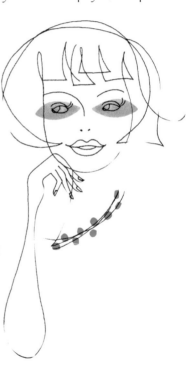

Confidently speaking

Confidence shows in all that you say, do, and feel. Don't worry that being confident will make you appear arrogant. Arrogance is a belief that you know more than other people. Confidence is when you know yourself! Confidence comes when you feel comfortable with who you are. It begins when you put your best foot forward with regards to dressing, hairstyle, makeup, defining your own style, and enjoying who you are. Being truly confident is knowing that you look and feel great in your own skin! What a wonderful feeling!

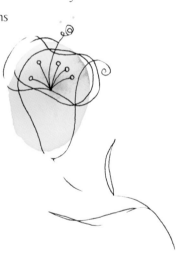

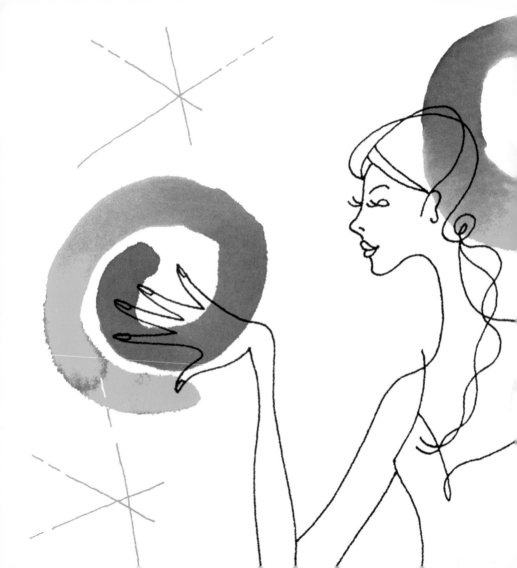

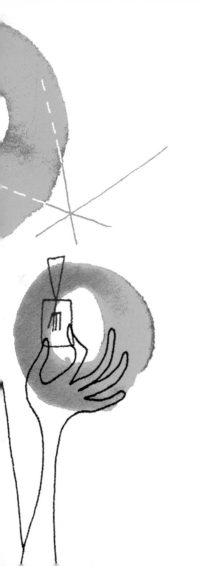

Chapter 4
Hands and feet

Footloose

Feet take such a beating. Put some spring into your step with this invigorating footbath treatment. Soak feet in warm soapy water. Mix one cup of granulated sugar and two tablespoons of almond or sesame oil. Rub into the feet and ankles for two minutes. Rinse, dry, and slip into some cotton socks. Leave socks on for at least two hours. Better yet, keep them on overnight. Feet will feel smooth and moisturized.

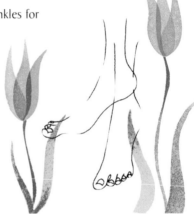

A step ahead

For the perfect home pedicure, keep in step. Begin by removing old polish and/or body oils from the toenails. Trim toenails and smooth edges with an emery board. Soak feet in a basin filled with warm water. Add one cup of scented bath salts along with some anti-bacterial soap. After soaking for ten minutes, rub foot, heel, and toe areas with a pumice stone to smooth out any rough spots. Coat cuticles with cuticle oil then push them back with an orange stick. Dry feet with a towel. Massage feet with a moisturizing cream until it is completely absorbed. Soak a cotton ball in polish remover and re-cleanse the toenails to remove any leftover cream. Apply a base coat. Follow with two coats of a wonderful, feel-good polish, and end with a shiny topcoat. Allow five minutes between coats to prevent smudging of polish. Wait at least one hour before putting on shoes or socks—flip-flops are perfect to wear as your toes dry.

Clean your plate

Nail plates that are stained and discolored from dark nail color polishes can benefit from a little nail plate cleaning. One way is to soak the nails in white vinegar for ten minutes. Rinse, dry, and apply cuticle oil. If stubborn stains persist, mix two tablespoons of household bleach and $\frac{1}{2}$ cup of warm water. Place nails in mixture for 15 minutes. Discoloration stains should be gone. Be sure to rinse well, pat dry, and slather on hand cream and cuticle oil to finish.

Manicure maintenance

One sure-fire way to maintain your manicure longer is to apply hand cream to your hands at least twice a day—if not more. Hydrating the hands will keep hangnails and cuticles in check. To keep nails looking freshly polished, apply a coat of topcoat every day. The topcoat will add days to the life of your manicure.

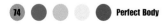

Lemon aid stand

To keep knees, elbows, and skin on the heels in the softest condition and free from discoloration, make some lemon "aid." Squeeze the juice from a lemon into two tablespoons of sugar. Apply the mixture to heels, elbows, and knees. Allow to work for two to three minutes. Gently rub off with a warm washcloth, pat dry, and add a dab of moisturizer. Areas will feel silky smooth and look more even in color.

No shave

To keep irritation at a minimum, it is best not to shave before swimming in a chlorinated pool, before a salt or mud treatment, or before a pedicure. Sunburned and extra dry skin should also deter you from shaving. If your moisturizer contains AHAs (alpha hydroxy acids) do not use the product right after shaving; it could cause burning or irritation.

 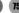

Beach baby

A walk along a sandy beach is a great way to strengthen and tone calves and legs. Running in and out of the waves is also good for the feet, since salt water has marine extracts and minerals which help soothe and smooth the skin. Plus, the salt water helps to gently exfoliate the feet and legs. So shed your shoes, and your cares, and start strolling.

Sands of time

To escape to the beach anytime—if only in your mind—enjoy this footprint exfoliation treatment. Mix $\frac{1}{2}$ cup of sand (found at craft and garden stores) with one tablespoon of sea salt and $\frac{1}{2}$ cup of olive oil in a bowl. Massage feet and legs with the mixture over a big basin. Rinse feet in slightly cool water to remove excess. Pat dry and enjoy your smooth feet!

Polish pointers

For the longest-lasting manicures, avoid "quick dry" polishes. While these five-minute wonders may save you drying time, you will more than make up for it with re-polishing. This extra work is due to "quick dry" polish's high acetone level. Acetone promotes drying, but at the expense of longevity. What good is saving time if it costs more time in the long run?

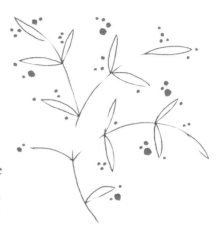

Opt for a regular polish and speed up drying time by applying a quick-drying spray to the nails after polishing, or try dipping the nails into ice water a few times.

Hands down

A perfect home manicure treatment begins by removing nail polish and/or oils from the nail bed by applying a polish remover. An easy way to remove nail polish is to soak a cotton ball with polish remover, place on the nail and hold in place for about ten seconds. The nail polish will become soft, allowing for an easier removal. File nails to desired shape and length with an emery board. (Metal nail files are too harsh, and cause the nail to weaken or crack.) Allow nails on each hand to soak in a bowl of anti-bacterial, soapy water for five minutes. Remove and dry hands. Clean gently under nails with a file. Apply cuticle oil and push cuticles back with an orange stick. Buff the nail beds with a nail buffer to create a smooth area on which to polish. Put a bit of polish remover on a cotton ball, and gently swipe each nail bed to remove any left over cuticle oil from the nail before polishing. Apply base coat. Add two coats of your favorite polish and finish with a topcoat to protect color and add shine. Allow at least five minutes between coats. Perfect every time!

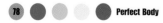

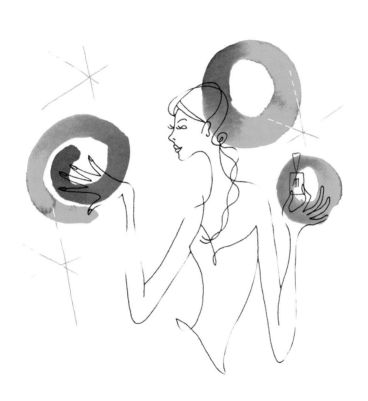

Painted lady

A beautiful pedicure and manicure can distract from other, less than perfect parts of the body. Be footloose and wild on toe polish, while keeping the fingernails a bit calmer. Because we use our hands so much, lighter colors help conceal chipping better than vibrant colors. Also, lighter colors detract attention away from the hands—especially helpful if hands are not in the best shape.

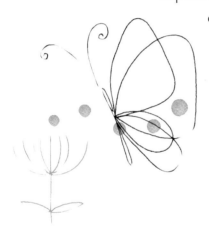

You're nailed

You are out of polish remover, your nails are totally unacceptable, and you have a major appointment in less than one hour in which your hands will definitely be on display. A quick fix remedy is to coat your nails, one hand at a time, with a clear base coat. Leave on for about ten seconds to allow the old nail polish to soften. Then press a tissue on the nail, pulling the tissue down toward the end of the nail to remove old polish in one swoop. If all of the old polish is not removed, apply the base coat again—wait just a couple of seconds and tissue it off. Nails are then ready to be repainted. Be sure to put polish remover on your shopping list, so that you won't be caught out again!

In a snap

To keep fingernails and the delicate cuticle skin healthy and hydrated, rub cuticle oil or vitamin E oil on them daily. Keep a bottle somewhere you can see it, and take just two minutes every day to do it. Vitamin E oil is excellent at protecting the nails from pool chlorine, so dab some on before you take a dip.

Accidental sun

Did you realize that on average, we get 23 hours of "accidental sun" each week? "Accidental sun" is sun that you may not even know you are getting as you walk to and from the car, stroll to the mailbox, or are stopped in sunny traffic with your hands on the steering wheel. You can even catch extra rays if your office or breakfast room is on the sunny side of the street. It all adds up. Sunscreen is not just for the beach—keep it in reach, daily, to keep the skin protected.

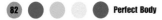

Hands on

Just like facial skin, our hands need special attention. As we age, the skin on the back of the hands wrinkles and loses elasticity, just as it does on the face. The fatty skin layers behind the epidermis become thinner; when the skin is pinched it does not return to its regular shape as quickly as it used to. Since our hands are usually on display, a good hand care routine is very important to keep hands looking their best.

Make it a habit to rehydrate your hands after you wash them, or as often as you can remember. Keep some hand cream, with added sunscreen, in your handbag and apply liberally throughout the day. After all, hands are the third area to show or deny age. (First is the face, and second is the neck.)

Defend and protect

Hands are not indestructible. Protecting them from the elements will keep them beautiful for years to come. When gardening, use gardening gloves to protect against yard chemicals and to keep dirt from lodging under the fingernails. Wear rubber gloves when cleaning or washing dishes, as soaps and detergents can be very abrasive on the skin. Keep a tube of hand cream next to the sink and remember to use it after you have washed the dishes. For an added bonus, slather on the hand cream before putting on rubber gloves. The heat from the water heats up the rubber gloves and allows for a better penetration of cream. Now you can consider chores a hand treatment!

Wonder where the yellow went

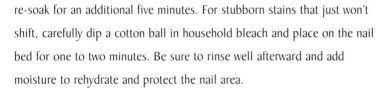

If nails are stained and yellowed from overdoing the darker nail colors, get them back to normal by soaking them in a solution of $\frac{1}{2}$ cup of grapefruit or lemon juice. Put nails in a small bowl of juice for five minutes and then rinse. If ugly stains persist, re-soak for an additional five minutes. For stubborn stains that just won't shift, carefully dip a cotton ball in household bleach and place on the nail bed for one to two minutes. Be sure to rinse well afterward and add moisture to rehydrate and protect the nail area.

Polish up your French

When it comes to nail trends, there is one look that never goes out of style: the French manicure. First hitting the Paris fashion scene in the mid '70s, the French manicure is even more popular than ever! After a base coat is applied, a coating of white polish is applied across the tips of the nail, creating a crisp, clean line where the nail edge is. Then a coating of either a sheer beige, or slightly pink nail polish is applied over the entire nail. Finally a top coat is applied to protect the nail and allow the manicure to last longer. The French manicure leaves your nails looking clean, fresh, and healthy—and matches anything you happen to be wearing.

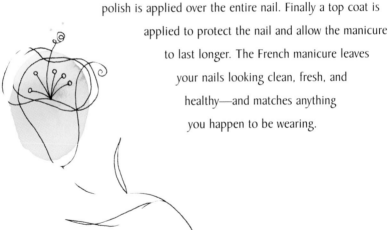

Professional nail tip

To keep your manicure lasting the longest after having a professional manicure, purchase the color that the technician applied to your nails. Touch-ups, should you need them, will be a breeze and you will be able to keep your professional manicure looking nicer for longer.

Seeing red

When visiting a professional manicurist or nail salon, be brave and experiment with your nail color. Don't just opt for the safe, barely-there colors—no doubt, you have a huge collection of similar nail colors collecting dust at home. Instead, take the opportunity to try a brighter, more vibrant tone. Burgandies, reds, pinks, and even mauves look great when applied neatly and make much more of a statement!

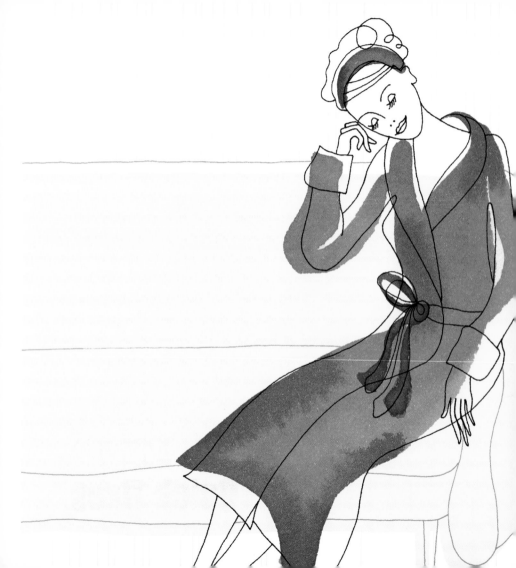

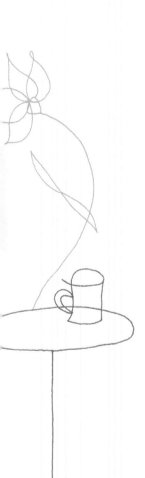

Chapter 5
Quick fixes

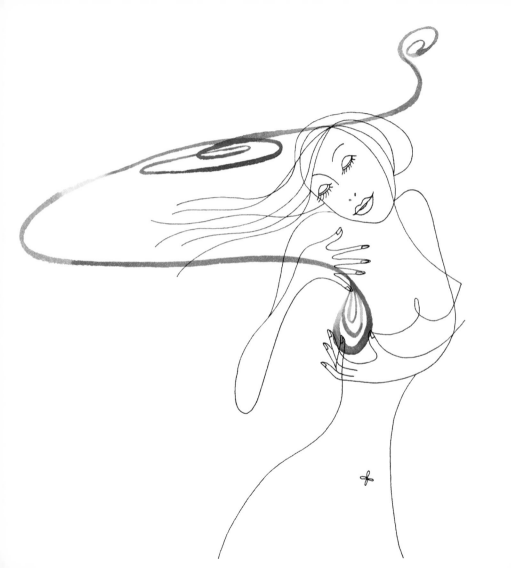

Backup plan

For backs that are prone to breakouts, rid the area of bacteria and dead cells and really deep clean by mixing two tablespoons of apple cider vinegar in a cup of warm water. Soak a washcloth in the mixture and gently cleanse the entire back area. Allow to dry. Do not rinse. Doing this treatment once a week should keep your back looking its best.

Break out of breakouts

Aloe vera juice detoxes as well as nourishes oily or acne prone backs, arms, and chests. Fill the bathtub with very warm water and add one cup aloe vera juice. Allow the water to fully cover the problem areas. Soak for ten minutes. Then take a washcloth, and pour aloe vera juice onto the cloth until it is saturated. Gently cleanse the area with the cloth. Immerse your skin once again in the tub and then pat dry.

Foot reviver

If your feet have walked the last mile and cannot go on, a foot soak is a fabulous reviver. But not just any foot soak. Combine three tablespoons of baking soda with two denture-cleansing tablets in a large basin. Soak the feet for ten minutes and rinse. Feet (and soul) will feel renewed, revived, and raring to go. Perfect after long workdays or day-long shopping excursions.

Feet detox

To soothe tired feet in a flash, try this trick. Apply Vaporub to clean, dry feet. Put on cotton socks and hop into bed. Vaporub is a decongestant that cools the skin and soothes aches and pains. When you awaken, your feet will feel ultra smooth and relaxed. This is a perfect item to keep in your travel bag for any extra walking that you might do whilst on vacation.

P. U.

Sometimes, no matter what, feet develop an unpleasant odor, in spite of cleansing routines. To refresh footsies in a short amount of time, soak feet for ten minutes in a mixture of two cups of brewed chamomile tea and three drops of peppermint. The chamomile will gently soothe and clean, while the peppermint sanitizes the feet. No need to rinse, simply pat dry, and apply a foot powder to

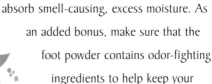

absorb smell-causing, excess moisture. As an added bonus, make sure that the foot powder contains odor-fighting ingredients to help keep your footsies fragranced—pleasantly!

Foot notes

To ease stress as well as tone the leg muscles, try these feats. While sitting down, practice picking up a wash cloth with your toes. Scrunch up your toes to pick up the cloth and lift it off the floor. Repeat ten times. Also try picking up marbles with the feet and dropping them into a bowl.

This exercise requires concentration, so banish all other thoughts from your mind for an instant de-stress session.

Turn down the heat

If hot weather makes you sticky, try adding a bit of baking soda to your body powder before applying. Baking soda absorbs excess moisture as well as odor. If your underarms have a tendency to stain the underarms of clothing, put a little baking soda over your deodorant to set and protect the garment.

Over exposed

While it goes without saying that sun exposure is bad for you, sometimes, no matter what precautions you take, the sun shines in. Here are some remedies to ease the pain and discomfort of overexposure:

✳ Mix $\frac{1}{2}$ cup of whole milk and one tablespoon of baking soda. Soak a washcloth in the mixture and gently pat on scorched areas.

✳ Mix two tablespoons of vinegar and one cup of water. Soak a washcloth in the mixture and place on the parched skin.

✳ Think pink. Calamine lotion works miracles on overdone skin. Smooth it on for instant, calming relief.

✳ For face overexposure, in addition to the sunshine cures above, gently massage the oil from an opened vitamin E capsule onto the skin to promote healing.

Leave the day behind

A quick fix after overworked, harried, excessive days is to take the day off of you by putting on a soft, oversized, luxurious spa-type bathrobe. Putting on the robe will signify leaving the day behind. It is the perfect uniform for snuggling in for the night or preparing for an evening out.

Chill out

When you are aching for a rubdown, but no masseuse is around, try this sure soother. Apply rubbing alcohol over any sore areas. As the alcohol evaporates, the cooling sensation will reduce soreness as well as calm the muscles and nerves. A perfect way to relax and de-stress after a busy day!

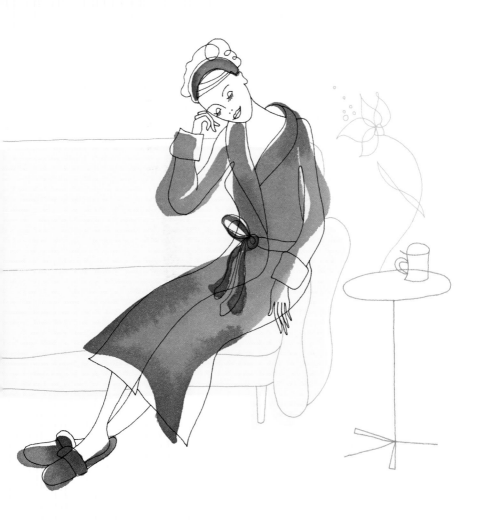

Banish the bloat

Sometimes no matter what
you do, the bloat gets you.
Tight rings, pants that
barely button—it's that
blah, bloated feeling. It
could be hormones or
just over-indulgent eating.
Whatever the cause, it needs
to go—now! A quick slim-down
drink that aids in fluid reduction is
a vegetable cocktail. Blend one cup
of cabbage, an apple, a few sprigs of
parsley, two carrots, and two stalks of celery in
a juicer. Sip on this bloat-reducing beverage for
a day or two. You will find that your clothes and
rings fit and all is now right with the world.

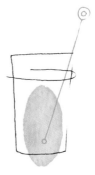

Exercise your options

As people have become more interested in keeping fit and exercising (which is excellent!), more and more of us are working up a sweat. With this extra activity, we are also showering more, and our skin is drying out as a result. If your skin is being affected by this increased cleansing, switch to a gentler body cleanser containing shea butter or milk proteins. Shea butter and milk products contain hydrating ingredients that help moisturize the skin upon contact. After drying off, slather on body lotion to keep skin hydrated. Be sure to keep travel sizes of body cleanser and lotion in your gym bag for cleaning on the go.

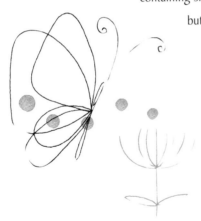

Leg relief

If dry, flaky skin on the legs has you kicking mad, relief has arrived. Before retiring, exfoliate legs. Then apply a facial mask to the legs. Allow to work for ten minutes, rinse, and pat dry. Slather on the most hydrating cream that you can find—the thicker, the better. Put on a pair of cotton leggings and wear to bed. In the morning your legs will glide out of bed feeling silky and ready to be exposed.

Innovative luxury

If high-end fragranced body lotions are out of your budget, make your own. Find a good, basic body moisturizer, and add a spritz or two of your favorite fragrance to your hand before applying the moisturizer as usual. You can also mist your fragrance on regular unscented talcum powder before applying, for a fresh and subtle scent.

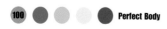

Outwit the ingrown

Ingrown hairs are painful, frustrating, and downright ugly. To keep yours to a minimum, gently exfoliate the affected area daily with a loofah, bath mitt, or bath sponge, while in the shower. By keeping the area free of extra dead skin cells, the hair shaft will remain open, allowing the hair to grow naturally, instead of being trapped underneath the skin.

New skin care products are on the market to aid in the reduction of ingrown hair. You can either roll them over the area, or apply them as a body moisturizer. The

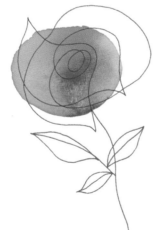

products contain ingredients that also help prevent the condition from reoccurring. Look for ingredients such as salicylic acid and alpha hydroxy acids to help end the problem.

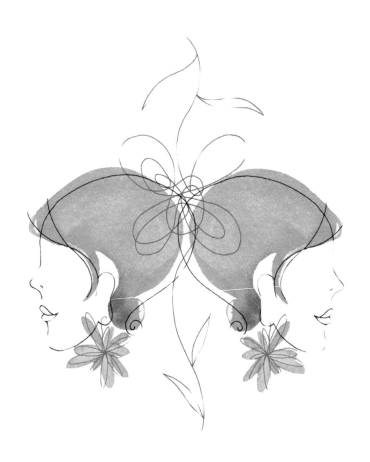

Ears to you

If you cannot bear to throw away inexpensive earrings that make your earlobes sore, try coating the posts and backs of the earrings with some clear, hypoallergenic nail polish. The coating of nail polish will form a barrier between your ears and the earring, making your sensitive skin less likely to react to the metal.

To be on the safe side, apply a second coating of the polish before attempting to wear the earrings. Be sure to allow your earlobes to completely heal before wearing troublesome earrings again—if at all. Fashion does have a price, but ask yourself—what is the real cost of inexpensive earrings? And is it worth it?

In a pinch

When you are absolutely, positively pooped, but have several more things on your to-do list, try this quick energy fix. Pinch the point on your hand between your thumb and pointer finger for two minutes. Change hands and repeat. This ancient acupressure point is the area that releases instant energy.

For really stubborn energy slumps, repeat once again on both hands. If that doesn't work—forget your to-do list and take a nap!

In the fast lane

To rev up your body in the morning—treat yourself to an energy shake. Blend together one banana, one cup of mineral water, one cup of low fat yogurt in your favorite flavor, and add one cup of your fruit du jour. Fruits that make excellent energy shakes are strawberries, peaches, oranges, and blueberries—either fresh or frozen will do just fine. Be sure to have this "wake-up" energy drink on an empty stomach to allow for the fastest vitamin and nutrient absorption.

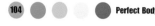

Banish body problems

The right essential oil can help your body banish some bothersome problems:

✳ Black pepper warms sore muscles. Sprinkle a few drops under the running bathwater before getting in.

✳ Neroli promotes healthy circulation and the scent relaxes at the same time.

✳ Mandarin oil eases fluid retention. Sprinkle five to seven drops in a very warm tub and allow the oil to help ease out the excess.

✳ Grapefruit essential oil alleviates muscle fatigue. Mix a few drops in a carrier oil or olive oil, and rub to ease the soreness.

Strike a pose

To make sure that you look your absolute best and allow your best side to show, do what the models do and strike a pose. Stand at a slight angle—between profile and straight ahead. This will accentuate your good curves and features while downplaying any less-than-perfect parts.

Undercover agent

Correctly fitting bras are your body's number one anti-aging agent. Studies show that 70 percent of us are wearing the incorrect bra size.

For your best figure, make an appointment with an expert bra fitter. Most department stores and boutiques have a resident bra fitter or schedule a visiting fitter several times throughout the year. The appointment takes about 15 to 20 minutes and the results of a properly fitted bra are dramatic! Not only can you take off ten pounds—but also five to ten years!

Did you know that as a B cup you carry about five to seven pounds on your breasts? C cups have about eight to 14 pounds and a D cup is carrying an average of 15 to 23 pounds! No wonder so many women are suffering from back problems. Get yourself measured today!

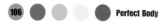

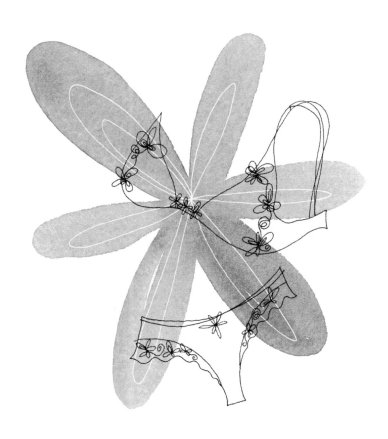

Susie Galvez

Armed with quick wit, years of professional experience, and more get-pretty tips than a beauty pageant coordinator, expert makeup artist, esthetician, and author Susie Galvez is dedicated to giving women tools to help them accept themselves and realize that each day is another chance to be beautiful.

Inspired by the thrill she gets from helping women rediscover beauty on a daily basis, Susie wrote the *Ooh La La! Effortless Beauty* series which includes *Ooh La La! Perfect Face, Ooh La La! Perfect Body, Ooh La La! Perfect Makeup,* and *Ooh La La! Perfect Hair.*

Susie is also the author of *Hello Beautiful: 365 Ways to Be Even More Beautiful, Weight Loss Wisdom: 365 Successful Dieting Tips,* and *InSPArations: Ideas, tips & techniques to increase employee loyalty, client satisfaction and bottom line spa profits.*

In addition to writing, Susie owns Face Works Day Spa in Richmond, Virginia. Face Works Day Spa has been featured in national and consumer magazines such as *Allure, Cosmopolitan, Elle,* and *Town and Country* as well as many trade publications including *Skin, Inc., Dermascope, Day Spa, Salon Today, Nails*

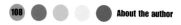

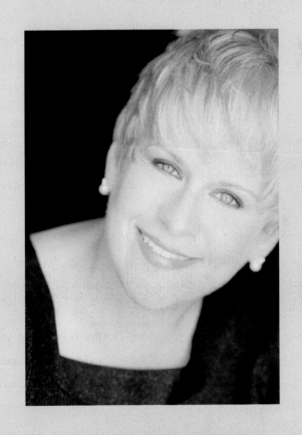

Plus, *Nails*, *Spa Management*, and *Les Nouvelles Esthetiques*. In April 2002, The Day Spa Association recognized Face Works as one of only 12 fully accredited day spas—out of 1,000 members—in the United States.

Susie is also recognized as one of the leading consultants in the spa industry, and is in high demand as a speaker at international spa conventions. She is a featured spokesperson for the beauty industry on radio and television programs and is a member of Cosmetic Executive Women, The National Association of Women Business Owners, and the Society of American Cosmetic Chemists.

You can contact Susie at www.susiegalvez.com or by visiting her beauty website at www.beautyatyourfingertips.com, where you will find even more ways to have Ooh La La moments! Be sure to sign up for your free spa-at-home tips!

Special appreciation

"Follow your bliss." Joseph Campbell

This book could not have been completed without the unwavering support and love from my very special friends. Thank you for allowing me to follow my bliss:

Dean Miller for keeping me on track and teaching me to actually enjoy exercising.

Audra Baca whose youthful spirit and turn of the word captured "me" on paper.

Dottie Dehart and Celia Rocks for their persistence in carrying my message out to the multitudes day after day.

Zaro Weil, friend and publisher, who entrusted me with her title.

To the superb massage and nail technician staff at Face Works Day Spa, who are responsible for creating the perfect bodies for our clients, Robin Payton, Karen Tucker, Monica Newton, Tamara Maxson, and Toni Richerson.

And lastly, but always first with me, thank you Tino Galvez who is truly the wind beneath my wings.

XOXO

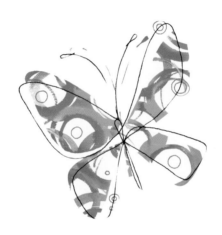